To ....

This Notebook is just for you!

From ....

Instagram: Creabooks
CREABOOKSPUBLISHINGS@GMAIL.COM

Made in the USA
Las Vegas, NV
16 November 2021

34559131R00068